"Dash Diet Cookbook For Beginners"

Discover Delicious Recipes to Manage Heart Diseases

Dr. Linda Wilson

Copyright © [2023] [Linda Wilson]

Table of contents

Introduction

The **"Dash Diet Cookbook For Beginners"** is your entryway to a healthier and more fulfilling existence.

This cookbook is intended to introduce you to the DASH (Dietary Approaches to Stop Hypertension) diet, a tried-and-true method of nourishing your body while lowering your risk of hypertension and other health issues.

In these pages, you'll embark on a culinary journey that not only delights your taste buds but also promotes overall well-being.

Whether you're new to the DASH diet or looking to refresh your culinary skills, this cookbook is your trusted companion.

We'll start with the basics, explaining the core principles of the DASH diet and guiding you through meal planning and preparation techniques.

You'll be equipped to create wholesome and nutritious dishes that fit seamlessly into your daily routine.

Discover an array of flavorful breakfasts to kickstart your day, salads and soups brimming with wholesome ingredients, and satisfying main courses that prove healthy eating can be truly delectable.

Delight in our selection of DASH-approved snacks and appetizers, along with sweet treats that won't compromise your health goals.

The DASH lifestyle isn't just about eating well; it's about embracing wellness as a whole.

That's why we've included bonus sections on fitness and exercise routines to complement your newfound culinary expertise.

Whether you're cooking for yourself or hosting a gathering, this cookbook provides options for every occasion.

Say goodbye to bland and restrictive diets and embrace the abundance of flavors and textures the DASH diet has to offer.

So get ready to embark on a journey of taste, nourishment, and well-being.

Let this cookbook be your guide as you take the first steps toward a healthier, happier you with the "Dash Diet Cookbook For Beginners." Let's savor the journey together!

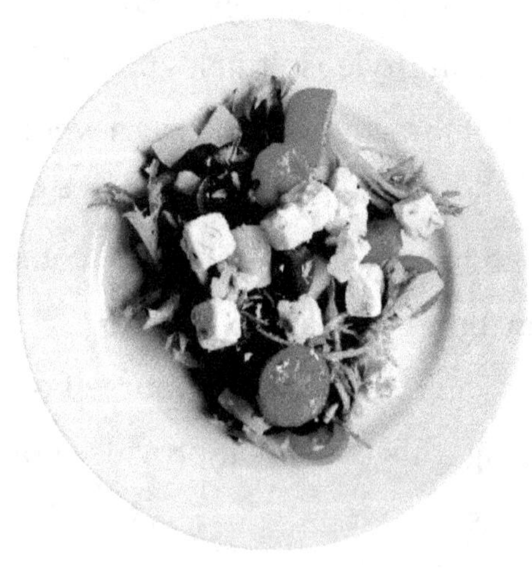

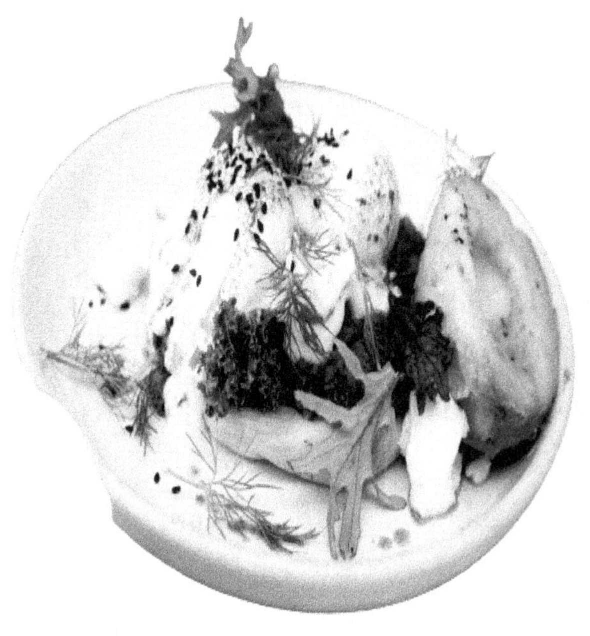

Chapter 1: The Basics of the DASH Diet

Welcome to the foundation of the DASH Diet, a healthful and balanced approach to eating that has garnered recognition for its effectiveness in promoting heart health, reducing hypertension, and fostering overall well-being.

In this chapter, we delve into the core principles of the DASH Diet, equipping you with essential knowledge to kickstart your journey towards a healthier lifestyle.

Understanding the DASH Diet

The DASH Diet, which stands for Dietary Approaches to Stop Hypertension, was developed by the National Heart, Lung, and Blood Institute (NHLBI) to combat high blood pressure.

However, its benefits extend far beyond that, making it a highly versatile and sustainable eating plan.

At its core, the DASH Diet emphasizes a balanced intake of nutrients, including fruits, vegetables, whole grains, lean proteins, and low-fat dairy.

By focusing on these food groups and minimizing sodium, saturated fats, and processed foods, you can enhance your heart health and overall wellness.

The DASH Diet Food Groups

1. Fruits and Vegetables: These colorful powerhouses are rich in vitamins, minerals, and antioxidants, which are essential for supporting your immune system and promoting cell health.

Incorporating a variety of fresh, frozen, or canned fruits and vegetables into your meals is key to meeting your nutritional needs.

2. Whole Grains: Replace refined grains with whole grains like brown rice, quinoa, oats, and whole wheat, as they contain fiber, which aids digestion and helps maintain steady blood sugar levels.

3. Lean Proteins: Opt for lean protein sources such as poultry, fish, legumes, tofu, and nuts, which provide essential amino acids and contribute to muscle repair and growth.

4. Low-Fat Dairy: Choose low-fat or fat-free dairy products to benefit from calcium and vitamin D while minimizing saturated fats.

5. Nuts, Seeds, and Healthy fats: These nutrient-dense sources of healthy fats, including monounsaturated and polyunsaturated fats, are beneficial for heart health when consumed in moderation.

reducing Sodium intake

Consuming too much sodium frequently results in high blood pressure.

The DASH Diet recognizes the importance of limiting sodium to maintain a healthy cardiovascular system.

By cutting back on added salt and avoiding highly processed foods, you can significantly reduce your sodium intake and better regulate your blood pressure.

Balancing Macronutrients

The DASH Diet strikes a harmonious balance of macronutrients: carbohydrates, proteins, and fats.

By moderating portions and choosing healthier options within each group, you can optimize your energy levels, support weight management, and promote overall vitality.

Tailoring the DASH Diet to Your Needs

One of the many strengths of the DASH Diet is its flexibility.

It can be adapted to accommodate various dietary preferences and needs, including vegetarian, vegan, or gluten-free diets. Whether you are an individual seeking to maintain a healthy weight, a fitness enthusiast, or someone looking to manage specific health conditions, the DASH Diet can be tailored to suit your lifestyle.

As you embark on this journey of health and wellness, keep in mind that the DASH Diet is not a quick fix but a sustainable way of eating. Gradual and consistent changes will lead to long-term benefits for your heart, body, and mind.

In the next sections of this cookbook, we'll delve further into practical tips for meal planning, preparation, and recipe ideas to bring the DASH Diet to life on your plate. Let's take the next step together and embrace the goodness of the DASH Diet for a healthier and happier you!

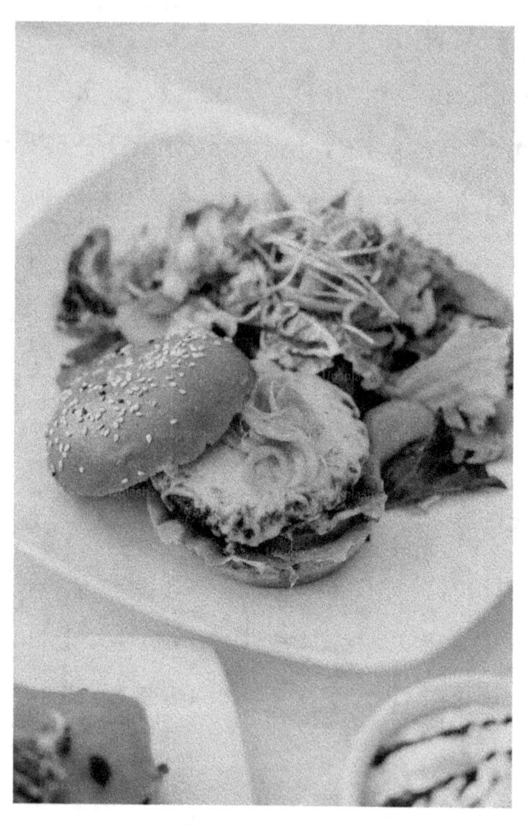

Chapter 2: Kickstarting Your DASH Journey: Meal Planning and Preparation

Congratulations on taking the first step towards embracing the DASH Diet as a way of nourishing your body and enhancing your well-being! In this chapter, we'll guide you through the essential aspects of kickstarting your DASH journey, from understanding meal planning to preparing nutritious and delicious dishes that align with the DASH principles.

The Power of Meal Planning

Effective meal planning is at the heart of a successful DASH journey.

By dedicating some time to thoughtful planning, you'll set yourself up for a week of healthy eating without feeling overwhelmed. Here's how to get started:

1. Assess Your Goals: Define your health and dietary objectives.

Whether you aim to lower your blood pressure, manage your weight, or simply improve your overall health, understanding your goals will shape your meal planning decisions.

2. Create a Weekly Schedule: Develop a weekly meal schedule, including breakfast, lunch, dinner, and snacks.

By having a plan in place, you'll be less likely to rely on unhealthy convenience foods or resort to last-minute decisions.

3. Explore DASH-Friendly Recipes: Look for an array of DASH-friendly recipes that resonate with your taste preferences.

 Aim for a balance of nutrient-rich ingredients and diverse flavors to keep your meals exciting and enjoyable.

4. **Shop Wisely:** Compile a shopping list based on your planned meals.

Focus on fresh produce, lean proteins, whole grains, and low-fat dairy.

Avoid impulse buying of processed snacks and sugary treats.

5. Prep Ahead: Spend some time prepping ingredients in advance to streamline your cooking during busy weekdays.

Wash, chop, and portion fruits and vegetables, and consider preparing larger batches of grains and proteins to use in multiple dishes.

Mastering DASH-Friendly Cooking

Now that you have your meal plan in hand, let's delve into the art of DASH-friendly cooking. Here are some essential guidelines to remember.

1. Flavor without Sacrifice: Experiment with herbs, spices, and aromatic ingredients to elevate the taste of your dishes without relying on excess salt or unhealthy fats.

2. Go Fresh and Seasonal: Whenever possible, choose fresh, seasonal produce.

Not only will this enhance the taste of your meals, but it will also provide you with a variety of nutrients.

3. Choose Lean proteins. Opt for lean cuts of meat, poultry, and fish, or explore plant-based protein sources like lentils, beans, and tofu. These options are rich in nutrients and lower in saturated fat.

4. Get Creative with Whole Grains: Embrace the versatility of whole grains like quinoa, barley, and farro.

These nutrient-dense alternatives add texture and flavor to your meals while contributing to better heart health.

5. Mindful Portions: Pay attention to portion sizes to ensure you're consuming balanced and appropriate amounts of each food group.

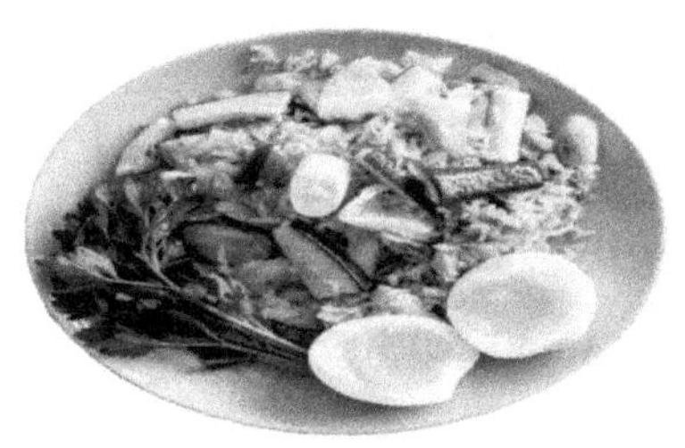

Embracing Meal Prep

Meal prep is a powerful tool to help you stay on track with your DASH Diet. Consider the following meal prep strategies:

1. Batch Cooking: Prepare larger quantities of certain recipes and freeze them in individual portions.

This way, you'll always have a healthy meal on hand, even on the busiest days.

2. Snack Smartly: Portion out nutritious snacks like cut fruits, vegetables, and nuts for easy access throughout the week.

3. Pre-portioned lunches: Prepare pre portioned lunches for work or school to avoid impulse purchases of less healthy options.

Remember, consistency is key to reaping the full benefits of the DASH Diet.

As you progress on your journey, you'll find that planning and preparation become second nature, leading to a more health-conscious and fulfilling lifestyle.

Stay tuned for the next chapters, where we'll explore a variety of flavorful breakfasts, wholesome main courses, and delightful DASH snacks and appetizers.

Let's continue this journey together, one nourishing meal at a time!

Chapter 3: Flavorful Breakfasts to Energize Your Day

Breakfast is the most important meal of the day, and on your DASH journey, it becomes an opportunity to kickstart your mornings with a burst of energy and wholesome goodness.

In this chapter, we present a delectable array of flavorful breakfast ideas that align with the DASH Diet principles, ensuring you start your day with a nutritious and satisfying meal.

1. Berrylicious Overnight Oats:

Indulge in the delightful combination of rolled oats, low-fat Greek yogurt, and a medley of fresh berries. Prepare this easy, make-ahead breakfast the night before and wake up to a delightful burst of flavor, antioxidants, and fiber that will keep you full until lunchtime.

2. Veggie-Packed Frittata:

Whisk together eggs, a splash of skim milk, and a colorful assortment of vegetables like spinach, bell peppers, and cherry tomatoes. Baked to perfection, this savory frittata provides a protein-packed start to your day while sneaking in a generous serving of veggies.

3. Avocado Toast with a Twist:

Upgrade your classic avocado toast by topping whole-grain bread with sliced avocado, a sprinkle of chia seeds, and a drizzle of extra virgin olive oil.

The creamy avocado, rich in healthy fats, paired with the crunch of chia seeds, makes for a satisfying and nourishing breakfast.

4. Nutty Banana Smoothie Bowl:

Blend together ripe bananas, unsweetened almond milk, and a spoonful of almond butter for a luscious and nutrient-dense smoothie. Pour it into a bowl and top with granola, sliced fruits, and a sprinkle of cinnamon to add texture and flavor to your morning routine.

5. Quinoa Breakfast Bowl:

Start your day with a protein-packed bowl of cooked quinoa, topped with fresh fruits, a dollop of low-fat yogurt, and a drizzle of honey. This wholesome breakfast will keep you feeling satisfied and energized throughout the morning.

6. Spinach and Feta Breakfast Wrap:

Wrap scrambled eggs, sautéed spinach, and crumbled feta cheese in a whole-grain tortilla for a portable and nutritious breakfast option. This hearty wrap provides a perfect blend of protein and greens to fuel your day.

7. DASH-Friendly Pancakes:

Enjoy a stack of fluffy, whole-grain pancakes made with mashed bananas, unsweetened applesauce, and a touch of cinnamon. Top with fresh berries and a drizzle of pure maple syrup for a delightful and guilt-free treat.

8. Chia Seed Pudding Parfait:

Combine chia seeds with unsweetened almond milk and let them soak overnight.

In the morning, layer the chia seed pudding with mixed berries and a sprinkle of nuts for a refreshing and nutrient-rich parfait.

9. Mediterranean Breakfast Plate:

Compose a breakfast plate with sliced tomatoes, cucumber, olives, and whole-grain pita bread.

Pair it with a soft-boiled egg and a serving of hummus for a Mediterranean-inspired breakfast that celebrates the goodness of wholesome ingredients.

10. Apple Cinnamon Baked Oatmeal:

Bake rolled oats, diced apples, and a dash of cinnamon for a comforting and flavorful breakfast.

This baked oatmeal can be prepared in advance and reheated for a quick and satisfying morning meal.

Energize your day with these delightful and nourishing breakfast options that celebrate the abundance of flavors and nutrients the DASH Diet has to offer.

The best part? Each recipe is designed to fuel your body, support your well-being, and promote a healthier, happier you.

Stay tuned for more mouthwatering DASH-approved dishes as we continue on this culinary adventure together!

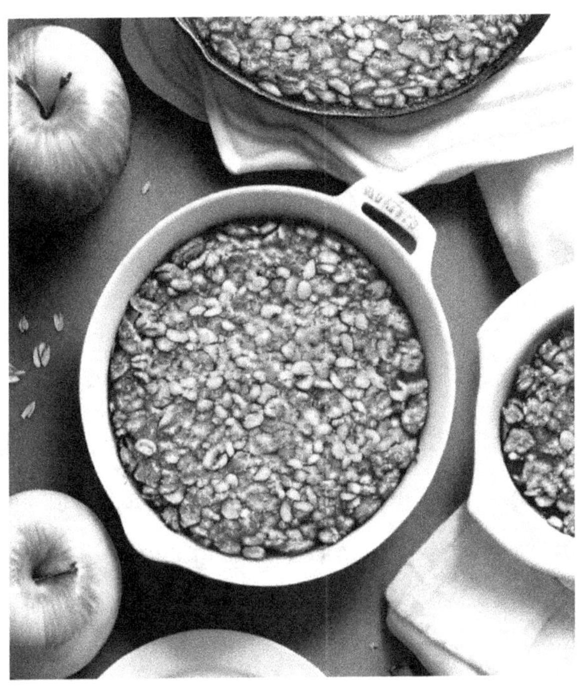

Chapter 4: Wholesome and Nutritious Salads and Soups

In this section, we investigate a dynamic universe of healthy and nutritious plates of mixed greens and soups that impeccably epitomize the substance of the Scramble Diet. Overflowing with a variety of varieties, seasons, and supporting fixings, these dishes provide a superb method for consuming a wealth of nutrients, minerals, and fiber while advancing heart wellbeing and, by and large, prosperity.

1. Garden New Quinoa Salad: Combine cooked quinoa with a mixture of new vegetables like cucumbers, cherry tomatoes, ringer peppers, and destroyed carrots.

Prepare with a light lemon vinaigrette and enhance with chopped spices for a reviving and protein-stuffed salad that will leave you feeling fulfilled and renewed.

2. Hearty Soup with Lentils and Vegetables: Stew lentils with various vegetables like onions, celery, and carrots in an exquisite vegetable stock.

Injected with fragrant spices and flavors, this good soup is both soothing and thick, making it an optimal choice for a feeding dinner.

3. Salad with Mediterranean Chickpeas: With a drizzle of balsamic vinaigrette, combine chickpeas, diced cucumbers, juicy cherry tomatoes, and feta cheese.

The flavor combinations in this salad, which is influenced by the Mediterranean, are delightful and highlight the benefits of plant-based protein and fresh produce.

4. Rich Tomato Basil Soup: Enjoy the velvety texture of a tomato soup made with fresh basil, garlic, and ripe tomatoes.

Utilizing low-fat milk or coconut milk rather than heavy cream keeps this soup light while safeguarding its delectable taste.

5. Barbecued Chicken Caesar Salad: Barbecue a chicken breast and serve it over a bed of fresh romaine lettuce.

Serve this classic salad with whole-grain croutons, a drizzle of Parmesan cheese, and a light Caesar dressing to satisfy your taste buds without jeopardizing your health goals.

6. Butternut Squash and Apple Soup: Broil butternut squash and sweet apples, then mix them into a smooth soup with a smidgen of warm flavors.

This soup, which is based on fall, is loaded with vitamins and antioxidants, making it a delicious and nourishing option for cooler days.

7. Salad with Edamame from Asia: Throw steamed edamame with destroyed cabbage, ringer peppers, and a lively ginger soy dressing. This salad is a magnificent combination of surfaces and flavors, providing an abundance of plant-based supplements.

8. Minestrone Soup with Entire Wheat Pasta: Enjoy the flavor of a traditional minestrone soup made with whole wheat pasta, white beans, and vegetables.

Offering a hearty meal that encourages a healthy diet, this Italian favorite is both filling and satisfying.

9. Roasted Beet and Goat Cheddar Salad: Combine creamy goat cheese, baby spinach, and candied walnuts with earthy beets that have been roasted until they are tender. Shower with a balsamic reduction for a plate of mixed greens that energizes your taste buds and commends the magnificence of regular fixings.

10. Sustaining Chicken Vegetable Soup:
Stew chicken stock with a grouping of brilliant vegetables, including zucchini, carrots, and green beans.

Add destroyed chicken for protein support, making a healthy and consoling soup that is ideally suited for any season.

These nutritious salads and soups support your efforts toward a healthier lifestyle by providing your body with essential nutrients and enriching flavors and textures. With each spoonful or forkful, you'll encounter the wizardry of healthy fixings, taking you closer to the delight of good wellbeing and prosperity. Remain tuned for additional feeding recipes as we proceed with our culinary experience with the Scramble Diet!

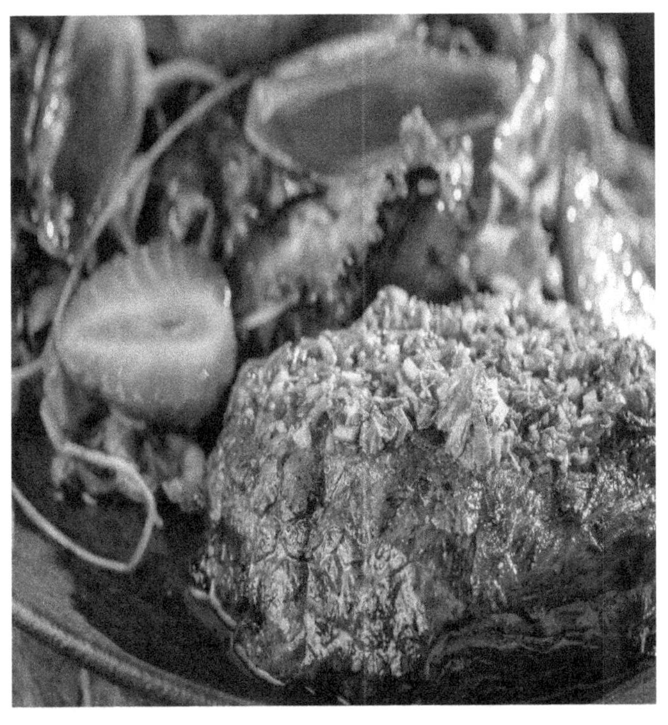

Chapter 5: Dash Diet–Friendly Recipes

1. Grilled Lemon Herb Chicken:

Ingredients:

chicken breasts without skin and bones

Citrus juice

Almond oil

minced garlic

Oregano, thyme, and rosemary are fresh herbs.

Pepper and salt

Preparation:

Lemon juice, olive oil, minced garlic, fresh herbs, salt, and pepper should all be combined to form a marinade for the chicken. Cook completely on the grill.

2. Quinoa Salad with Veggies:

Ingredients:

Quinoa Cherry tomatoes, diced, half red bell peppers, diced, diced red onions, freshly minced fresh parsley, and lemon juice
Almond oil
Pepper and salt

Preparation:

As directed on the package, prepare the quinoa. Cooked quinoa, diced veggies, fresh parsley, lemon juice, olive oil, salt, and pepper should all be combined in a bowl. Stir thoroughly, then plate.

3. Baked Salmon with Dill Sauce:

Ingredients:

Filets of salmon

Greek yogurt, fresh dill, and

Dillon mustard

citric acid

powdered garlic

Add pepper and salt.

Preparation:

On a baking sheet, arrange the salmon filets. In order to produce the sauce, combine the chopped dill with the Greek yogurt, Dijon mustard, lemon juice, garlic powder, salt, and pepper.
Spread the sauce over the salmon, then bake it until it's fully done.

4. Mediterranean Chickpea Salad:

Ingredients:

a can of chickpeas, halved cherry tomatoes, drained and rinsed cucumber, pitted and sliced red onion, finely chopped feta cheese, and olive oil
white wine vinegar
Dry oregano
Add pepper and salt.

Preparation:

Combine chickpeas, cherry tomatoes, cucumber, olives, red onion, and feta cheese in a big bowl. Red wine vinegar and olive oil should be drizzled on.
Add salt and pepper, along with the dried oregano. Serve after a good toss.

5. Turkey and Vegetable Stir-Fry:

Ingredients:

turkey that is lean

florets of broccoli

slice of a carrot

Snow peas and chopped red bell pepper

salt-free soy sauce

Olive oil, chopped Ginger, and grated Garlic

Preparation:

Cook ground turkey with minced garlic and ginger in olive oil in a wok or large skillet over high heat.

Stir-fry the added vegetables until they are soft.

Over brown rice, add low-sodium soy sauce for flavoring.

6. Spinach and Mushroom Egg White Omelette:

Ingredients:

Whites of eggs
leaves of spinach
Sliced onions and mushrooms
(Optional) Low-fat cheese
Add pepper and salt.

Preparation:

The egg whites are whisked with salt and pepper. Sliced onions and mushrooms should be cooked until soft in a nonstick pan.
Then, add the spinach leaves and the egg whites.
Cook the omelet just until it sets. Before serving, fold the omelet and top with low-fat cheese, if preferred.

7. Lentil and Vegetable Soup:

Ingredients:

the red lentil

chopped carrots, celery, onion, and onion, diced

mashed up tomatoes

Bay leaves in a vegetable broth

Cumin Paprika

Add pepper and salt.

Preparation:

Cook celery, carrots, and onions in a large pot until they are tender.

Sea salt, pepper, bay leaves, red lentils, smashed tomatoes, vegetable broth, cumin, and paprika.

Simmer for a while to cook the lentils and thicken the soup.

8. Grilled Shrimp Skewers:

Ingredients:

Deveined and peeled zucchini, sliced red onion,
and large shrimp
the cherry tomato
Lemon zest and olive oil
chopped fresh basil
Add pepper and salt.

Preparation:

Shrimp, cherry tomatoes, red onion chunks,
and zucchini slices are all skewered together.
Olive oil should be drizzled over the dish before
adding the lemon zest, chopped basil, salt, and
pepper.
The shrimp should be grilled until they are
fully cooked and pink.

9. Roasted Brussels Sprouts with Balsamic Glaze:

Ingredients:

trimming and halving Brussels sprouts

Extra virgin olive oil

the vinegar of balsam

The honey Dijon mustard

peppermint oil

Both salt and pepper

Preparation:

Add salt, pepper, and olive oil to the halved Brussels sprouts. Bake until the food is crispy and slightly tender.

Honey, Dijon mustard, garlic powder, balsamic vinegar, and a small bowl. Roasted Brussels sprouts should be covered with the glaze before serving.

10. Baked Sweet Potato Fries:

Ingredients:

sliced sweet potatoes served as fries

Paprika and olive oil

powdered garlic

Add pepper and salt.

Preparation:

The oven should be heated to 425°F (220°C).
Combine olive oil, paprika, garlic powder, salt,
and pepper with the sweet potato fries.
They should be layered evenly on a baking pan.
Fries should be crispy and golden brown after
20 to 25 minutes of baking, flipping halfway
through.

**Enjoy these delicious and healthy Dash
Diet Lounge recipes!**

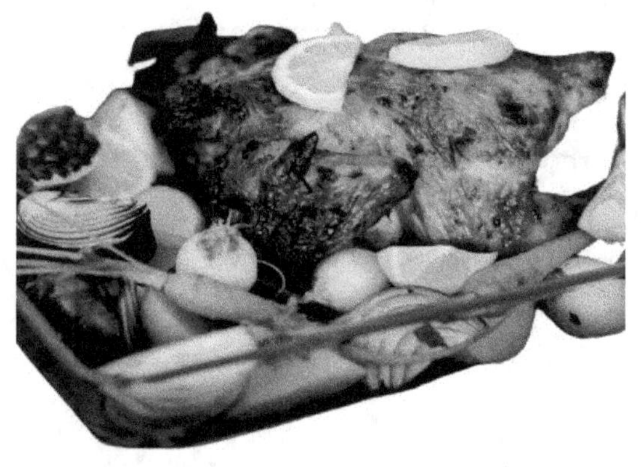

Chapter 6: Satisfying and Savory Main courses

Welcome to the core of your Scramble Diet culinary experience, the domain of fulfilling and flavorful principal courses that will leave you feeling fed and content.

In this part, we present a different determination of delicious dishes, painstakingly created to commend the kinds of entire food varieties while sticking to the standards of the Scramble Diet.

1. Prepared Lemon Spice Salmon:

Marinate new salmon filets in a fiery mix of lemon, garlic, and new spices, then, at that point, heat until delicate and flaky.

This omega-3-rich dish tempts your taste buds as well as supports heart wellbeing and general prosperity.

2. Stir-Fry with Veggies:

Stir-fries are a delicious and adaptable way to show off a variety of vibrant vegetables.
Throw broccoli, chile peppers, snap peas, and tofu in a light pan-fried food sauce for a speedy and nutritious fundamental course that overflows with flavor.

3. Stuffed Ringer Peppers:

Lean ground turkey, brown rice, diced tomatoes, and a dash of cumin make a flavorful filling for vibrant bell peppers.
Prepared flawlessly, these stuffed peppers make for a healthy and outwardly shocking dish.

4. Grilled Chicken from Her Bed:

Barbecue delicious chicken breasts marinated in a variety of new spices, olive oil, and lemon juice.
This flavorful, squishy main course is packed with protein and is both filling and light, showcasing the simplicity of healthy ingredients.

5. Vegan Chickpea Curry:

Stew chickpeas and a variety of vegetables in a rich tomato-based curry sauce.

This plant-based curry, infused with an exotic mix of spices, promises to be a satisfying and filling meal.

6. Zucchini Noodles with Pesto Sauce:

Making your own basil pesto sauce and spiraling the zucchini into strands that resemble noodle shapes.

Top with cherry tomatoes and toasted pine nuts for an invigorating and low-carb option in contrast to customary pasta dishes.

7. Lean Hamburger and Vegetable pan-fried food:

Saute lean pieces of meat with a grouping of brilliant vegetables, for example, carrots, chime peppers, and snow peas.

Throw in a light soy sauce and ginger dressing for a protein-pressed pan sear that fulfills your desires for Asian-propelled flavors.

8. Spinach and Mushroom Stuffed Chicken Bosom:

Stuff chicken breasts with a combination of sauteed spinach, mushrooms, and feta cheese. Heated until delicate, these stuffed chicken breasts are a brilliant mix of surfaces and flavors, ideal for unique events or weeknight meals.

9. Mediterranean Eggplant Baked:

Layer cuts of eggplant with tomatoes, onions, and a sprinkle of feta cheese.

Heated until delicate and brilliant, this Mediterranean-propelled dish exhibits the magnificence of healthy fixings and captures the substance of the Scramble Diet.

10. Quinoa and Dark Bean Enchiladas:

Roll cooked quinoa and dark beans in corn tortillas, then cover them in an energetic enchilada sauce and a sprinkle of softened cheddar.

Heated flawlessly, these enchiladas offer a protein-rich and fulfilling primary course that is ideally suited for social occasions or family suppers.

These filling and savory main courses, each intended to nourish your body and elevate your dining experience, celebrate the richness of flavors and textures.

Continue your journey toward improved health and well-being by embracing the DASH Diet's culinary artistry.

Remain tuned for additional culinary enjoyments as we investigate the Scramble Diet's healthy and tasty world together!

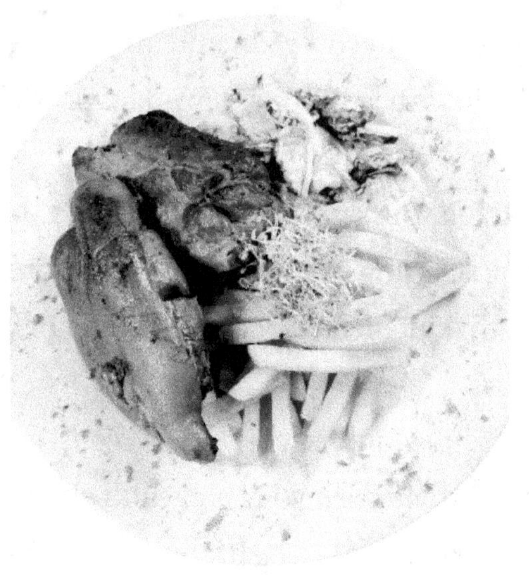

Chapter 7: Delicious DASH Diet Snacks and Appetizers

In the realm of the DASH Diet, snacking and appetizers need not be dull or compromising. In this chapter, we invite you to savor the art of wholesome snacking with a pleasurable selection of mouthwatering snacks and appetizers that align impeccably with the principles of the DASH Diet.

These treats aren't only satisfying but also brimming with essential nutrients to fuel your body and support your well-being.

1. Guacamole with Veggie Dippers
Indulge in delicate and scrumptious guacamole made with ripe avocados, minced tomatoes, red onions, and a splash of lime juice.
Brace it with a multifarious variety of brick vegetable ladles like carrot sticks, cucumber slices, and bell pepper strips for a stimulating and nutritional snack.

2. Greek Yogurt Parfait: Subcategories low-fat Greek yogurt with fresh berries, a sprinkle of granola, and a drizzle of honey for a protein-rich and naturally candied parfait.

This pleasurable treat offers a balance of textures and flavors, making it an excellent choice for a quick breakfast or noon pick-me-up.

3. Hummus and Whole Wheat Pita Chips

Dip into the satiny virtuousness of manual hummus made with chickpeas, tahini, bomb juice, and garlic.

Serve it with whole wheat pita chips for a satisfying and fiber-rich snack that is perfect for amusement or a single indulgence.

4. Caprese Skewers Thread cherry tomatoes, fresh mozzarella balls, and basil leaves onto rustic skewers for a pleasurable and visually appealing appetizer.

Mizzle with balsamic glaze for a burst of pungent flavor that elevates this classic combination.

5. Crunchy Roasted Chickpeas: Roast chickpeas with a sprinkle of your favorite spices until crisp and golden.

These scrumptious and protein-packed roasted chickpeas offer a guilt-free alternative to traditional snacks, satisfying your craving for crunch without compromising your health pretensions.

6. Cucumber and Tuna mouthfuls Top cucumber slices with a nugget of tuna salad made with canned tuna, Greek yogurt, minced celery, and a gusto of dill.

These light and refreshing mouthfuls provide a balance of protein and vegetables, making them ideal for a light lunch or appetizer.

7. Stuffed Mini Bell Peppers Fill halved mini bell peppers with an admixture of quinoa, black sap, minced tomatoes, and a sprinkle of trash.

Ignited until tender and golden, these stuffed peppers are both lovable and nutritious, making them a megahit at any gathering.

8. Fresh Fruit Kabobs Thread a multitude of various fresh fruits, such as strawberries, grapes, pineapple, and melon, onto skewers for a vibrant and vitamin-packed snack.
Serve with a side of low-fat yogurt for a pleasurable and stimulating treat.

9. Zesty Cilantro-Lime Shrimp Blend Marinate cooked shrimp in a salty mix of cilantro, lime juice, and a hint of chili.
Serve the shrimp blend with avocado slices and a side of whole-grain crackers for a savory and satisfying appetizer.

10. Smoked Salmon and Cucumber
Mouthfuls Subcaste smoked salmon on cucumber slices and top with a nugget of light cream and fresh dill.

These elegant and nutritional mouthfuls are perfect for special occasions or a sophisticated noon snack.

With these pleasurable gusto Diet snacks and appetizers, you can embrace the joy of conscious eating while nourishing your body with the virtues of whole foods.

Elevate your snacking experience with these tasteful treats, and stay tuned for further culinary alleviations as we continue our disquisition of the wholesome world of the DASH Diet together!

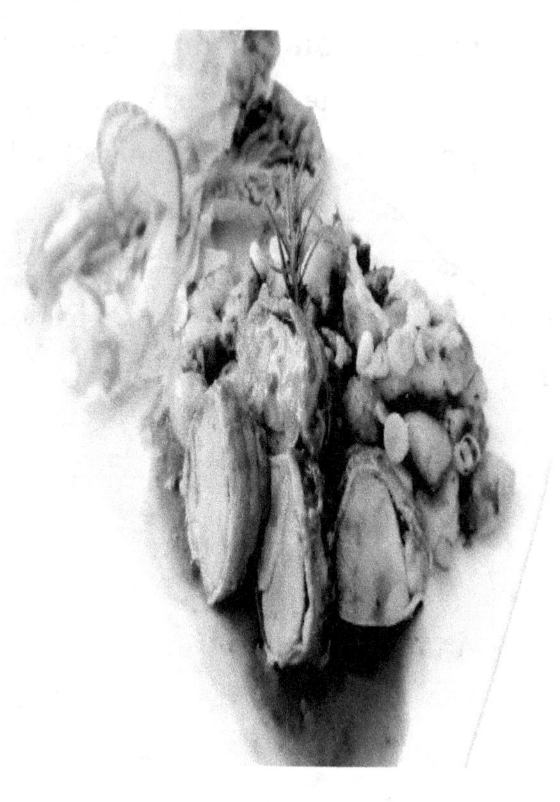

Chapter 8: Sweet Indulgences with a Healthy Twist

Who says enjoying desserts must be an indulgence? In this section, we welcome you to relish the specialty of sweet guilty pleasures with a sound bend as we present a brilliant choice of treats that adjust impeccably to the standards of the Scramble Diet.

These divine manifestations fulfill your sweet tooth as well as feed your body with healthy fixings, demonstrating that you can have your pastry and eat it as well!

1. Berry Chia Seed Pudding:

Join chia seeds with unsweetened almond milk and a bit of unadulterated maple syrup, then, at that point, layer it with a blend of new berries.

This velvety and supplement-rich chia seed pudding offers a virtuous pastry that is wealthy in cell reinforcements and fiber.

2. Dull Chocolate-Plunged Natural Product Mixture:

Liquefy dull chocolate and plunge an arrangement of new natural products like strawberries, bananas, and kiwi cuts.

The dark chocolate's rich flavor supplements the pleasantness of the organic products, making a delightful treat that fulfills your sweet desires while giving you fundamental nutrients and minerals.

3. Heated Apples with Cinnamon and Nuts:

Center and heat apples until delicate, then fill them with a combination of slashed nuts, cinnamon, and a shower of honey.

This warm and fragrant pastry offers an encouraging twist on the exemplary heated apple while adding a portion of sound fats and fiber.

4. Banana-Oat Treats:

Crush ready-made bananas and blend them in with moved oats, a sprinkle of cinnamon, and a small bunch of dark chocolate chips.

Prepared flawlessly, these chewy and normally improved treats are a magnificent treat for virtuous extravagance.

5. Frozen Yogurt Berry Bark:

Spread low-fat Greek yogurt on a material-lined baking sheet, then disperse a grouping of new berries on top.

Freeze until firm, and break it into pieces for an invigorating and low-calorie frozen treat that is ideally suited for warm days.

6. Peanut Butter Banana Frozen Yogurt:

Mix frozen bananas with a spoonful of regular peanut butter until smooth and velvety.

This delicious and sans-dairy "frozen yogurt" offers a fantastic and righteous option in contrast to conventional frozen yogurt, making it an optimal choice for a sweet treat.

7. Oats and Raisin Energy Nibbles:

Join rolled oats, raisins, honey, and a spot of cinnamon, then, at that point, structure the blend into reduced-down balls.

These energy nibbles have a characteristic pleasantness, making them ideal for fulfilling your sweet desires between feasts.

8. Scaled-down Lemon Poppy Seed Biscuits:

Prepare smaller than usual biscuits with entire wheat flour, poppy seeds, and an eruption of lemon zing.

These tart and superb treats are segment controlled, making them an extraordinary choice for a virtuous guilty pleasure.

9. Vanilla Berry Smoothie:

Mix low-fat milk, vanilla concentrate, and a blend of new berries into a rich and normally sweet smoothie.

This invigorating and supplement-stuffed refreshment is ideally suited for a fast and sustaining sweet or bite.

10. Caramelized Banana Cuts:

Sauté banana cuts in a bit of coconut oil until caramelized and brilliant.

These sweet and caramel-like banana cuts are ideal for garnishing yogurt, oats, or getting a charge out of all by themselves as a healthy treat.

With these sweet extravagances and a solid contort, you can enjoy the delight of pastries while supporting your body with the decency of whole and nutritious fixings.

Embrace the craft of careful extravagance and investigate the awesome universe of Run Diet sweet treats.

Remain tuned for more culinary motivation as we proceed with our excursion of healthy and tasty pleasures together!

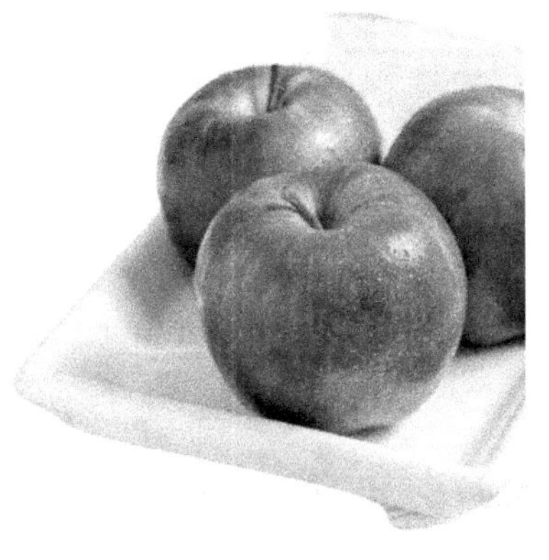

Chapter 9: DASH Diet Drinks and Refreshments

Extinguish your thirst and renew your faculties with a reviving turn, all as one with the standards of the Scramble Diet.

In this part, we dive into the universe of Run Diet beverages and rewards, offering you a heavenly cluster of drinks that hydrate as well as support your body with healthy fixings.

1. Citrus-implanted water:

Raise your hydration game by imbuing water with cuts of citrus natural products like oranges, lemons, and limes.

This normally seasoned water is an invigorating and cell-reinforcement-rich choice that urges you to hydrate throughout the day.

2. Green Tea with Mint and Honey:

Brew green tea and add a couple of new mint leaves and a shower of honey for a relieving and reviving beverage.

This fragrant mix offers a delicate caffeine boost alongside the potential medical advantages of green tea cell reinforcements.

3. Berry Ecstasy Smoothie:

Mix a blend of fresh or frozen berries with low-fat Greek yogurt and a sprinkle of almond milk.

This lively and supplement-pressed smoothie is a magnificent method for enjoying the regular pleasantness of berries while supporting your well-being objectives.

4. Coconut Water Boost:

Taste the normally hydrating coconut water, either all alone or mixed with a sprinkle of pineapple or mango juice.

This tropical-roused reward gives electrolytes and a bit of regular pleasantness, making pursuing it an optimal decision after an exercise.

5. Cucumber and Lemon Detox Water:

Join cut cucumbers, lemon wedges, and a couple of branches of mint in water for a detoxifying and empowering drink.

This mixed water helps with hydration as well as adding an eruption of flavor and a hint of spa-like style to your daily schedule. 6. Chilled,

6. Home-grown Hibiscus Tea:

Mix hibiscus tea and chill it over ice for a lively and tart drink.

Hibiscus tea is rich in cell reinforcements and is accepted to have possible cardiovascular advantages, making pursuing it a fitting decision for a Scramble Diet-motivated reward.

7. Chia Seed Lemonade:

Blend chia seeds with freshly squeezed lemon juice and water, and allow it to sit until the chia seeds form a gel-like surface.

This fiery and fiber-rich lemonade offers an extraordinary twist while providing fundamental supplements.

8. Mango Tango Smoothie:

Mix ready-made mango lumps with low-fat milk or non-dairy choices, alongside a bit of vanilla concentrate.

This tropical joy captures the quintessence of summer, offering a normally sweet and velvety treat.

9. Shimmering Water with Berries and Spices:

Consolidate shimmering water with a small bunch of new berries and a couple of crushed mint leaves.

This bubbly and outwardly engaging beverage adds a bit of class to any event while keeping you hydrated and revived.

10. Cinnamon-Flavored Hot Chocolate:

Warm up with some hot chocolate made with unsweetened cocoa powder, low-fat milk, and a sprinkle of cinnamon.

This comfortable and consoling drink offers a bit of extravagance with a solid twist.

With this Run Diet beverage and rewards, you can hoist your refreshment decisions while supporting your body with the integrity of normal fixings.

Embrace the delight of hydration and investigate the lively universe of flavors that the Scramble Diet brings to the table.

Remain tuned for more culinary motivation as we proceed with our excursion of healthy and tasty enjoyments together!

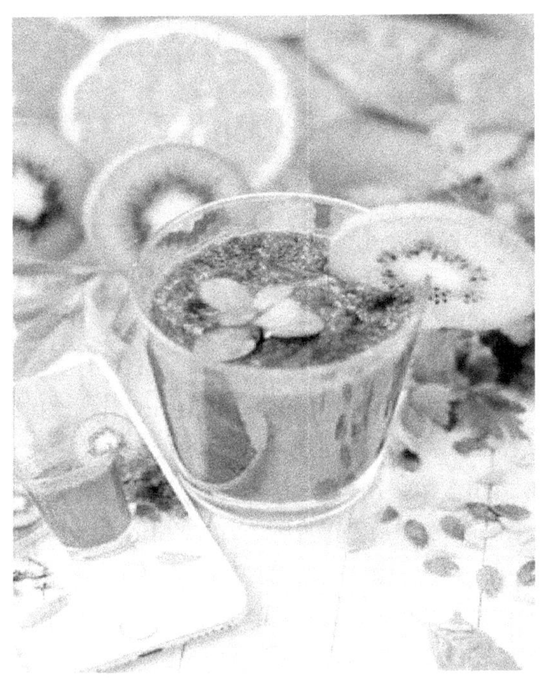

Chapter 10: DASH Diet for Special Occasions

Embracing the DASH Diet doesn't mean you have to sacrifice enjoyment on special occasions.

In fact, this chapter is dedicated to showcasing how the DASH Diet can seamlessly integrate into your celebrations, offering delectable dishes that are both wholesome and indulgent. Whether it's a birthday, holiday, or any moment worth celebrating, these special occasion recipes will make your gatherings memorable while staying true to the principles of the DASH Diet.

1. Roast Turkey with Herb Quinoa Stuffing:

For your festive feasts, consider a succulent roast turkey paired with a quinoa stuffing infused with fragrant herbs.

This balanced and flavorful combination caters to both tradition and health, providing a protein-rich centerpiece alongside a nutrient-dense stuffing.

2. Festive Grilled Vegetable Platter:

Create an eye-catching platter featuring an assortment of grilled vegetables like zucchini, bell peppers, and eggplant.

Arrange them artistically and serve with a balsamic glaze or yogurt-based dip for a vibrant and nutritious appetizer.

3. Cranberry-Almond Brussels Sprouts:

Elevate the classic Brussels sprouts side dish by adding toasted almonds and dried cranberries. This sweet and nutty medley complements the natural flavors of the Brussels sprouts, making it a perfect accompaniment to your special occasion meal.

4. Spinach and Feta Stuffed Mushrooms:

Fill large mushrooms with a mixture of sautéed spinach, crumbled feta cheese, and aromatic herbs.

Baked until golden, these stuffed mushrooms offer a delectable and elegant appetizer that's sure to impress your guests.

5. Herbed Salmon Fillet:
For an elegant entrée, present a baked salmon filet seasoned with a blend of fresh herbs and lemon zest.
The result is a dish that's both visually appealing and rich in heart-healthy omega-3 fatty acids.

6. Roasted Beet and Goat Cheese Salad Tower:
Construct a tower of roasted beet slices, goat cheese, and mixed greens drizzled with a balsamic reduction.
This artistic and flavorful salad adds a touch of sophistication to your special occasion table.

7. Dark Chocolate Raspberry Tart:
Indulge in a dark chocolate raspberry tart made with a whole grain crust and a velvety dark chocolate filling.
Topped with fresh raspberries, this dessert provides a rich and satisfying conclusion to your celebratory meal.

8. Berry and Mint Mocktail:

Craft a refreshing mocktail by muddling fresh berries and mint leaves with sparkling water. Garnish with additional berries and a sprig of mint for a vibrant and alcohol-free option that's perfect for toasting.

9. Herb-Infused Sparkling Lemonade:

Create a memorable and herb-infused sparkling lemonade by mixing freshly squeezed lemon juice with sparkling water and a hint of rosemary or thyme.

This aromatic and fizzy drink adds a touch of elegance to your special occasion.

10. Fruit Parfait Dessert Bar:

Set up a dessert bar featuring a variety of fresh fruits, low-fat Greek yogurt, and granola.

Allow your guests to create their own fruit parfaits, offering a customizable and health-conscious dessert option.

With these DASH Diet-inspired recipes for special occasions, you can celebrate with flavorsome dishes that prioritize health without compromising on taste.

Elevate your gatherings and create lasting memories as you showcase the versatility and deliciousness of the DASH Diet. Stay tuned for more culinary inspiration as we continue our journey of wholesome and flavorful delights together!

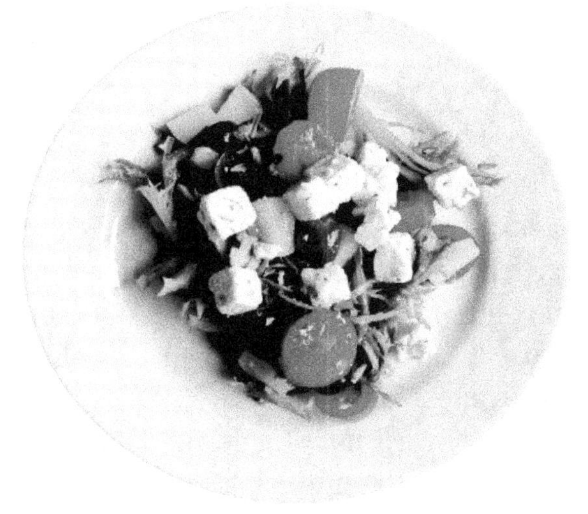

Chapter 11: Embracing the DASH Lifestyle: Tips for Long-Term Success

Progressing to the Dash (Dietary Ways to Stop Hypertension) way of life isn't just about keeping a bunch of guidelines; it's an excursion towards further developed wellbeing, imperativeness, and prosperity.

In this part, we'll investigate fundamental tips to assist you with embracing the Scramble way of life and guarantee long-term progress as you continue looking for a better and more healthy lifestyle.

1. Slow Movement:

Embrace the Scramble way of life with a slow methodology.

Begin by integrating Run-endorsed food sources and recipes into your eating regimen, bit by bit. This assists your sense of taste in acclimating to new flavors while forestalling sensations of limitation.

2. Adjusted Eating:

Center around adjusted feasts that integrate various supplement-rich food varieties.

Mean to incorporate lean proteins, entire grains, a lot of leafy foods, and sound fats in your day-to-day diet.

This approach upholds heart wellbeing as well as gives supported energy over the course of the day.

3. Careful Segments:

Practice careful eating by focusing on segment sizes.

Utilize more modest plates and bowls to assist with controlling portion sizes, and pay attention to your body's cravings and completion prompts.

Over the long haul, this propensity can prompt more careful and fulfilling dinners.

4. Hydration Propensities:

Remain hydrated by drinking water over the course of the day.

Choose water over sweet drinks, and consider implanting your water with cuts of citrus, cucumber, or spices for an invigorating turn. Appropriate hydration is fundamental for overall wellbeing and can supplement your Scramble way of life.

5. Savvy Nibbling:

Pick supplements with thick bites that line up with the Scramble standards.

Keep various solid choices close by, like new natural products, crude vegetables, Greek yogurt, and nuts.

These snacks provide fundamental supplements as well as help forestall reveling in less solid decisions.

6. Standard Active work:

Integrate standard active work into your daily schedule.

Whether it's lively strolling, running, cycling, or yoga, finding exercises you appreciate can add to your general prosperity and support your Scramble way of life objectives.

7. Cooking at Home:

Preparing feasts at home permits you to have full control over the fixings you use.

Explore different avenues regarding well-disposed recipes, spices, and flavors to make tasty dishes that make it simple to keep up with your new way of life.

8. Mind-Body Association:

Practice pressure-reducing methods like reflection, profound breathing, or care. Overseeing pressure is a fundamental piece of the Scramble way of life, as it can decidedly affect circulatory strain and general wellbeing.

9. Social Help:

Draw in your loved ones in your Scramble process. Share feasts, recipes, and encounters to establish a strong and supportive climate. Having an organization of individuals who comprehend and support your objectives can have a huge effect.

10. Consistency and Tolerance:

Recollect that the Scramble way of life is a drawn-out responsibility.

Show restraint toward yourself and shine a spotlight on progress as opposed to flawlessness.

Reliably making better decisions will prompt progressive and supportable upgrades in your wellbeing and prosperity.

By embracing these tips and coordinating them into your day-to-day schedule, you're putting yourself in a position for long-haul accomplishment with the Dash way of life. Each step you take carries you closer to accomplishing your wellbeing objectives and partaking in the advantages of a decent and feeding lifestyle.

Remain committed, remain enlivened, and progress forward with this satisfying excursion towards a better and more joyful you.

Chapter 12: Bonus Section: Fitness and Exercise Routines for Enhanced Results

Accomplishing ideal wellbeing and prosperity through the Dash (Dietary Ways to Stop Hypertension) way of life goes beyond sustaining your body with healthy food varieties.

Supplement your Scramble process with a wellness and workout schedule that upgrades your outcomes, reinforces your cardiovascular framework, and supports your general health. In this reward area, we'll investigate viable wellness systems and workout schedules custom-made to synergize with Run standards.

1. Cardiovascular Molding:

Take part in customary cardiovascular activities to support your heart's wellbeing. Exercises like lively strolling, running, swimming, and cycling hoist your pulse and advance better dissemination, adjusting impeccably with the Scramble objective of keeping up with sound circulatory strain.

2. Stop-and-go aerobic exercise (HIIT):

Integrate HIIT exercises into your everyday practice to boost calorie consumption and work on cardiovascular wellness.

These short explosions of extreme activity followed by brief periods of rest are time-effective and can be customized to your wellness level.

3. Strength-Preparing:

Coordinate strength preparation practices utilizing body weight, opposition groups, or free loads.

Reinforcing your muscles upholds your digestion, bone wellbeing, and, in general, actual capability, adding to a balanced wellness schedule.

4. Yoga and Adaptability:

Practice yoga or extend your schedule to improve adaptability, equilibrium, and unwinding.

Yoga supplements the Scramble way of life by advancing pressure reduction and care, the two of which contribute to cardiovascular wellbeing.

5. High-intensity aerobics:

Join cardiovascular activities, strength training, and bodyweight practices in a circuit design.

This approach keeps your exercise drawing in and varied, supporting by and large wellness and assisting you with remaining roused.

6. Dynamic Way of Life:

Integrate active work into your day-to-day practice.

Use the stairwell, walk or bicycle for little excursions, and stand or move around during stationary errands.

These little lifestyle changes add to your general day-to-day development and energy consumption.

7. Utilitarian Activities:

Integrate utilitarian developments that mirror genuine exercises.

These activities work on your capacity to perform regular errands easily and with certainty, upgrading your personal satisfaction.

8. Bunch Wellness Classes:

Join a bunch of wellness classes like dance, heart-stimulating exercise, or turning to mix it up and add social commitment to your gym routine and daily schedule.

Practice with others can support inspiration and assist you in remaining focused.

9. Careful Development Practices:

Investigate careful development exercises like yoga or Pilates.

These practices center around body mindfulness, balance, and controlled developments, supporting your physical and mental prosperity.

10. Progress and Transformation:

Consistently reconsider your wellness routine and make changes in accordance with your challenge.

Steadily increase the force, term, or intricacy of your exercises to keep seeing improvement over the long haul.

By integrating these wellness and exercise techniques into your Dash way of life, you're creating a comprehensive way to deal with wellbeing and prosperity.

Similarly, as the Dash Diet sustains your body from the inside, a well-planned wellness routine supports your actual strength, perseverance, and cardiovascular wellbeing. Embrace this reward segment as a significant asset to enhance your outcomes and lift your excursion towards ideal wellbeing and essentialness.

Keep in mind that each step you take towards a more dynamic and adjusted way of life carries you closer to a better and more joyful you.

Conclusion:

As we reach the end of this enriching culinary and lifestyle exploration, we hope you've discovered the true essence of the DASH (Dietary Approaches to Stop Hypertension) lifestyle—a journey towards vibrant health, wellness, and a harmonious relationship with food.

Throughout this book, we've embarked on a flavorful odyssey, uncovering the delights of nourishing recipes, mindful eating, and holistic well-being.

The DASH Diet isn't just a collection of dietary guidelines; it's a philosophy that celebrates the synergy between wholesome foods, mindful choices, and a balanced lifestyle.

We've dived into a realm of vibrant vegetables, succulent proteins, heart-healthy fats, and nourishing grains, crafting meals that please both the palate and the body.

Our recipes have showcased how every bite can be a joyful step towards better health, supporting your cardiovascular system, promoting weight management, and fueling your vitality.

However, the DASH journey goes further than the kitchen.

It's a path that promotes awareness, exercise, and a thorough comprehension of your body's requirements.

The DASH principles can be incorporated into your daily life in a variety of ways, from mindful eating to stress management.

We now understand how a comprehensive fitness program enhances your outcomes and adds a further level of holistic wellbeing to your life.

As you close this book, remember that the DASH lifestyle is a path paved with nutritious choices, mindful indulgences, and an unwavering commitment to your health.

Each step you take, each nourishing meal you savor, and each moment of mindful awareness bring you closer to a state of vibrant well-being. Embrace the knowledge you've gained and let it guide you towards a healthier, happier you.

May the flavors, insights, and inspirations you've discovered within these pages continue to be a source of guidance, motivation, and joy as you navigate your own unique DASH journey.

Remember, the true essence of the DASH lifestyle lies not only in its delicious dishes but also in the positive impact it has on your body, mind, and soul.

Here's to your continued health, vitality, and a life enriched by the nourishing embrace of the DASH way.

Cheers to your well-being and the extraordinary journey ahead!

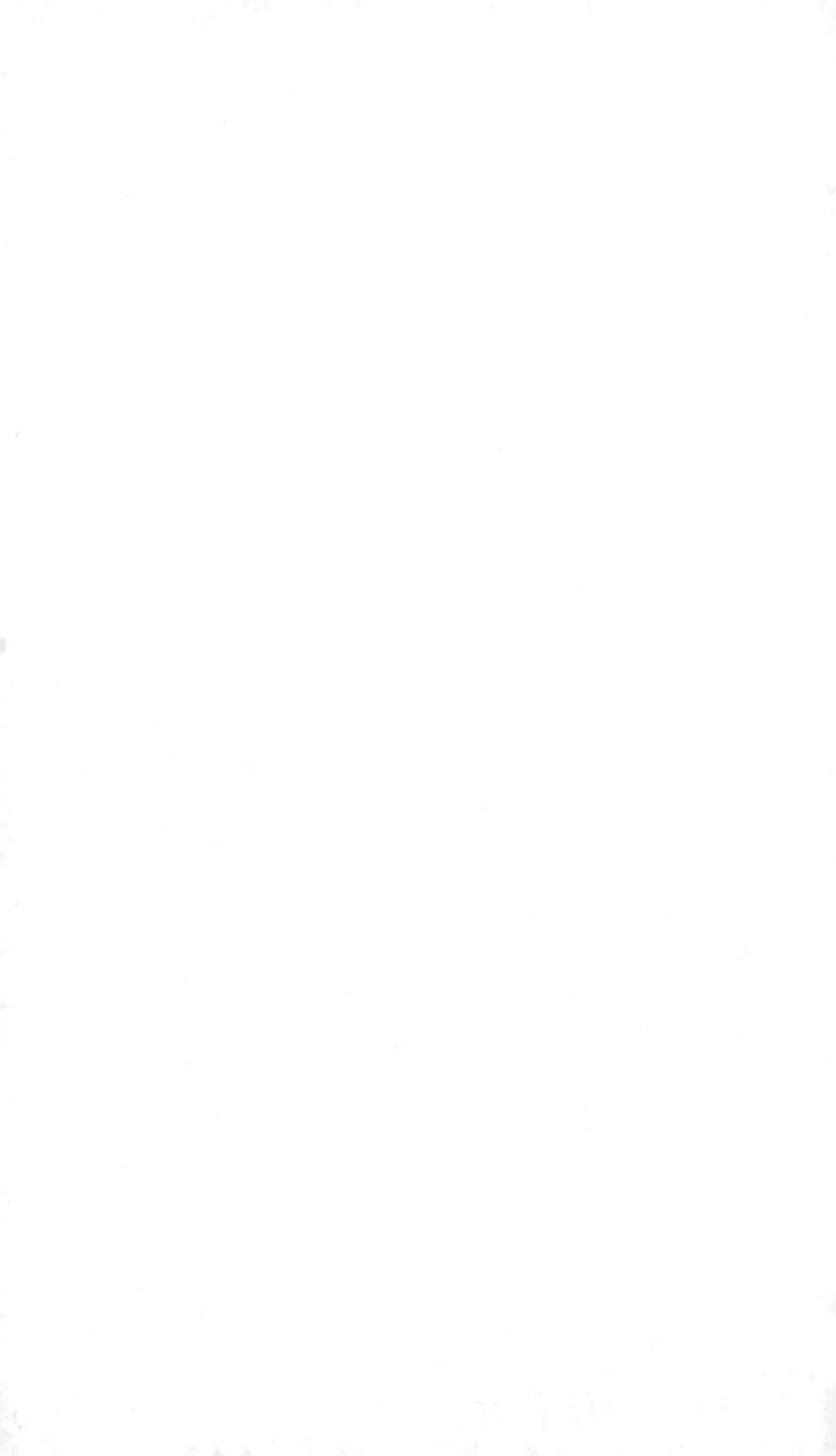